Camping Cookbook for Beginners

Affordable, Quick and Easy Camping Recipe Collection

America Camping Recipes

2

Contents

Spanish Skillet Tilapia 7

Herb Blackened Trout 10

Ginger and Lime Salmon 12

Baby Potato and Green Beans with Mozzarella "En Papilotte" 14

Gremolata Swordfish Skewers 16

Tofu Skewers with Spicy Peanut Sauce 18

Marinated Mushroom Kabobs 20

Creamy Grilled Potato Salad 22

Baby Gem Lettuce with Balsamic & Goat Cheese................................... 24

Balsamic Glazed Veggie Kabobs 26

Romaine Salad with Bacon & Blue Cheese 28

Potato Salad with Bacon Vinaigrette 30

Artichokes with Harissa-Honey Dip.. 32

Cumin Chili Potato Wedges... 34

Chili Con Carne 36

Hodge Podge 37

Campfire Chicken and Dumplings 39

Tomato Chickpea Soup 41

Spiced Lentil Soup 43

Chicken Stew Recipe 45

Barbeque Stew Packet 47

Tin Foil Stew.. 48

Wild Rice Soup 51

Fast Goulash.. 53

A Mean Three-Bean Salad.. 55

Mashed Potatoes 57

All Fruit Salad 58

All in One Burger and Sides 59

Amarillo Steak...60

Antipasta Dip 62

Arkansas Potatoes 63

Asian Marinade..64

Apricot Pork Chops 65

Bacon Burgers..66

Burger and Beans 68

Chuck Steak Stew...69

Cowboy Steak Packets..71

Ham, Asparagus and Potatoes..72

Ham and Pineapple 73

Ham and Swiss...74

Hamburger and Veggies 75

Oriental Chicken 76

Spicy Jerk Wings 78

Chicken in the Garden 80

Lemon Barbecued Chicken 82

Italian-Style Chicken 84

Chicken with Mushrooms..86

Tropical Chicken 88

Chicken Salad on a Bun..90

Ranch Chicken Pouches 91

Retro Baked Mac and Cheese...93

Jazzy Spanish Torta..95

Jumble-sale Jambalaya 97

Stuffed Cabbage Osijek Style 99

Papa's Chicken Paprikash.. 101

Faint-worthy Stuffed Eggplant 103

Messy Moussaka 105

Polenta Derventa 108

Lazy Lasagna with Ground Beef or Vegetables........................... 109

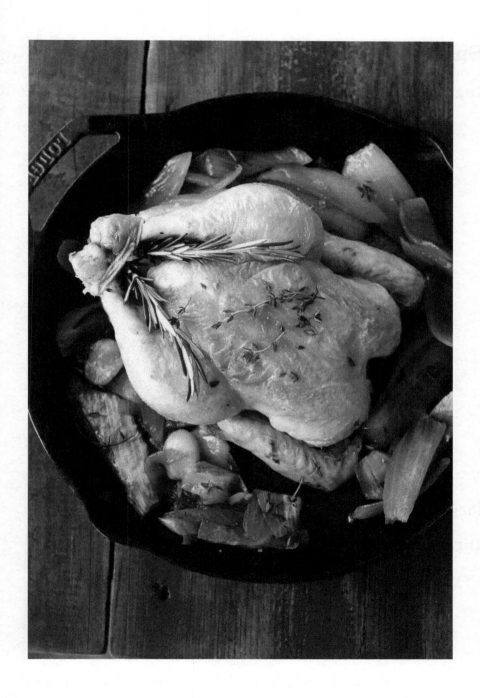

Spanish Skillet Tilapia

Ingredients:

- 4 tilapia fillets
- 3 tbsp. olive oil
- 2 tomatoes, chopped
- 1 red bell pepper, sliced
- 1 medium red onion, sliced
- 1/3 cup garlic tomato sauce
- 3 garlic cloves, minced
- 1/3 cup olives, pitted and halved
- 1 ½ tbsp. capers, rinsed and drained
- 1 tbsp. jalapeno peppers, chopped
- ¼ cup chicken stock
- 1 ¼ oregano
- Salt, to taste
- Pepper, to taste

Preparation: 10 minutes | Cooking: 10 minutes | Servings: 4

Directions:

1. Heat the oil in the skillet.
2. Pour in the chopped tomatoes, sliced bell peppers, and onion.
3. Season with salt and stir.
4. Reduce the heat to medium, cover with the lid and cook for 4 minutes.

5. Next, add the minced garlic, olives, capers, jalapeno peppers, chicken stock and tomato sauce.
6. Season the vegetables again with oregano, pepper and salt, and stir.
7. Sprinkle the filets with salt and pepper.
8. Place on top of the sauce and toss over the top of the fish.
9. Cover the fish and cook for 6 minutes.
10. **Remove from the stove.**
11. **Serve immediately and enjoy.**

Nutrition: Calories 129, Total Fat 2.7 g, Saturated Fat 0.9 g, Polyunsaturated Fat 0.6 g, Monounsaturated Fat 1 g, Cholesterol 57 mg, Sodium 56 mg, Potassium 380 mg, Total Carbohydrate 0 g, Dietary fiber 0 g, Sugar 0 g, Protein 26 g

<u>6</u>

Herb Blackened Trout

Ingredients:

- 6 trout fillets
- 1 ¼ tbsp. paprika
- 2 tsp. dry mustard
- 1 tsp. cayenne pepper
- 1 tsp. ground cumin
- 1 tsp. white pepper
- 1 tsp. black pepper
- 1 tsp. dried thyme
- 1 tsp. salt
- ¾ cup unsalted butter, melted
- ¼ cup unsalted butter, melted

Preparation: 20 minutes | Cooking: 10 minutes | Servings: 4

Directions:

1. Combine the paprika, dry mustard, cayenne pepper, cumin, black pepper, white pepper, thyme and salt into a small bowl. Set aside.
2. Heat the skillet on high heat.
3. In a shallow bowl, pour the ¾ cup butter. Dip the fillets in the butter.
4. Sprinkle with the spice mixture on both sides.
5. Set the fillets into the pan, leaving room.

6. Pour 1 tsp. butter over each fillet.

7. Cook for 2 minutes or until the fish has a charred look.

8. Turn the fish over and repeat the process.

9. Remove from the heat.

10. **Serve immediately and enjoy.**

Nutrition: Calories 383.5, Total Fat 21.2 g, Saturated Fat 3.2 g, Cholesterol 120.7 mg, Sodium 399.0 mg, Potassium 1,172.9 mg, Total Carbohydrate 2.9 g, Dietary Fiber 1.9 g, Sugars 0.4 g, Protein 43.9 g

Ginger and Lime Salmon

Ingredients:

- 4 (6-oz) salmon or tuna steaks, skin on
- 1 fresh lime (sliced)

For marinade:

- 1½ tablespoons soy sauce
- 1 tablespoon olive oil
- 4 garlic cloves, crushed
- 2 teaspoons ginger, peeled and grated
- 1½ teaspoons sesame oil
- ¼ teaspoon red pepper flakes
- ½ teaspoon sugar

Preparation: 40 minutes | Cooking: 15 minutes | Servings: 4

Directions:

1. Place the fish inside a sealable bag, and add marinade ingredients. Mix well to coat the fish completely.

2. NOTE: Raw seafood should be handled with care. Make certain not to reuse anything that touches the raw fish without thoroughly cleaning it first.

3. Allow fish to marinate for 30 minutes. Occasionally turn the fish in the bag to make sure they are evenly coated. Remove fish from marinade. Save the rest of the marinade.

4. Place a sheet of heavy-duty aluminum foil on the grill over the fire. Make sure the grill is set at the highest setting. Spray the sheet with cooking oil. Place fish, skin side down, on the foil sheet, then onto the grill, but not over a direct flame. Place thin lime slices over the top of the fish. Periodically baste with marinade.

5. Grill for 5-6 minutes per each ½ inch of the salmon's thickness. It should be done when the flesh flakes easily with a fork.

6. When ready, the fish should easily peel away from skin. Pair well with Baby Potatoes and Green Beans recipe (see next recipe).

Nutrition: Calories 277.4, Total Fat 7.4 g, Saturated Fat 1.1 g, Cholesterol 64.4 mg, Sodium 52.9 mg, Potassium 626.2 mg, Total Carbohydrate 30.7 g, Dietary Fiber 0.2 g, Sugars 28.4 g, Protein 23.4 g

Baby Potato and Green Beans with Mozzarella "En Papilotte"

Ingredients:

- 4 cups baby potatoes, washed and quartered
- 3 tablespoons pesto (jarred)
- ½ pound fresh green beans, washed and trimmed
- Salt and pepper, to taste
- 8 oz. mozzarella, diced

Preparation: 10 minutes | Cooking: 25 minutes | Servings: 4 to 6

Directions:

1. In a large bowl, mix potatoes and green beans with pesto.
2. Season the vegetables with salt and pepper to taste.
3. Make 4 aluminum foil packet sheets. Spray one side of each sheet with cooking oil spray.
4. Place a quarter of the vegetables on each foil sheet and close to form the packets.
5. Place directly on the white coals, grilling for about 20 minutes or until potatoes are soft.
6. Turn the packets over after 10 minutes.
7. Open foil packets and add cheese.
8. Cook 2-3 minutes more without closing the packet and placing them on the grill to melt and lightly color the cheese.

9. To serve, this dish accompanies fish dishes like the Ginger and Lime Salmon perfectly.

Nutrition: Calories 168.1, Total Fat 7.4 g, Saturated Fat 1.1 g, Cholesterol 0.0 mg, Sodium 1,177.9 mg, Potassium 606.2 mg, Total Carbohydrate 24.4 g, Dietary Fiber 5.0 g, Sugars 1.1 g, Protein 3.3 g

Gremolata Swordfish Skewers

Ingredients:

- 1 ½ lb. skinless swordfish fillet
- 2 teaspoons lemon zest
- 3 tablespoons lemon juice
- 1/2 cup finely chopped parsley
- 2 teaspoons garlic, minced
- 3/4 teaspoon sea salt
- 1/4 teaspoon black pepper
- 2 tablespoons extra-virgin olive oil, plus extra for serving
- 1/2 teaspoon red pepper flakes
- 3 lemons, cut into slices

Preparation: 20 minutes | Cooking: 10 minutes | Servings: 4

Directions:

1. Preheat griddle to medium-high.
2. Combine lemon zest, parsley, garlic, 1/4 teaspoon of the salt, and pepper in a small bowl with a fork to make gremolata and set aside.
3. Mix swordfish pieces with reserved lemon juice, olive oil, red pepper flakes, and remaining salt.
4. Thread swordfish and lemon slices, alternating each, onto the metal skewers.

5. Grill skewers 8 to 10 minutes, flipping halfway through, or until fish is cooked through.
6. Place skewers on a serving platter and sprinkle with gremolata.
7. Drizzle with olive oil and serve.

Nutrition: Calories 333, Sodium 554 mg, Dietary Fiber 0.5g, Fat: 16g, Carbohydrates 1.6g Protein 43.7g

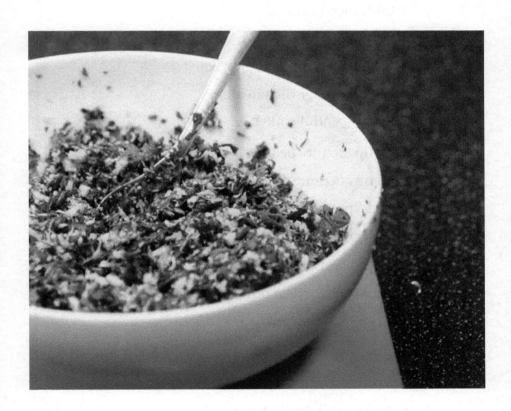

Tofu Skewers with Spicy Peanut Sauce

Ingredients:

For the grilled tofu skewers:

- 1 package extra-firm tofu, drained and pressed for 30 minutes or longer
- 2 tablespoons soy sauce
- 2 tablespoons water
- 1 tablespoon honey
- 1/2 teaspoon smoked paprika
- 1/2 teaspoon garlic powder

For the spicy peanut sauce:

- 1/2 cup creamy peanut butter
- 1/4 cup coconut milk
- 2 tablespoons soy sauce
- 2 tablespoons lime juice
- 1 tablespoon Sriracha
- 1/4 teaspoon garlic powder

Directions:

1. Cut the pressed block of tofu into 8 sticks.
2. Add the tofu, soy sauce, water, honey, smoked paprika, and garlic powder to a sealable plastic bag, seal, and toss to coat.
3. Refrigerate for a minimum of 1 hour or 24 hours before grilling.

4. Mix together all of the spicy peanut sauce ingredients in a small mixing bowl; set aside or refrigerate until needed.

5. Before grilling, pour the marinade into a bowl to use as a baste.

6. Thread the tofu onto metal skewers lengthwise.

7. Preheat the griddle to medium-high heat.

8. Grill the skewers for 10 to 15 minutes, turning as needed until char marks form on each side; baste with the leftover marinade often as they cook.

9. Serve hot with the spicy peanut sauce on the side for dipping.

Nutrition: Calories 138, Sodium 315 mg, Dietary Fiber 1.3g, Fat 10.6.g, Carbohydrates 7.8g, Protein 5.7g

Marinated Mushroom Kabobs

Ingredients:

- 1 punnet white button mushrooms, whole
- 1 green pepper, deseeded and cut into 2-inch pieces
- 1 yellow pepper, deseeded and cut into 2-inch pieces
- 1 onion, cut into 2-inch pieces
- 1-pint cherry tomatoes

For the marinade:

- 1/4 cup olive oil
- 2 cloves garlic, minced
- 1 lemon, juiced
- 1/2 teaspoon dried oregano
- 1/2 teaspoon sea salt

Preparation: 10 minutes | Cook time: 10 minutes | Servings: 4

Directions:

1. Arrange vegetables on metal skewers in an alternating pattern.
2. Place on a baking sheet or piece of aluminum foil.
3. Whisk together the marinade ingredients in a small mixing bowl and pour over skewers; turn skewers to coat well.
4. Preheat a grill to medium heat and cook 4 to 5 minutes on both sides until charred.
5. Remove kabobs to a serving tray and enjoy!

Nutrition: Calories 173, Sodium 243 mg, Dietary Fiber 4.2g, Fat 13.2.g, Carbohydrates 16.1g, Protein 2.7g

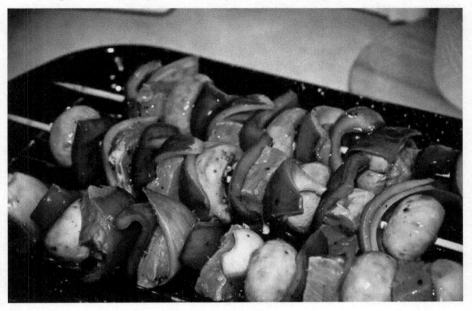

Creamy Grilled Potato Salad

Ingredients:

- 2 (1.5 lb.) bags baby white potatoes
- Non-stick cooking spray

For the dressing:

- ½ cup mayonnaise
- 1 tablespoon sour cream
- 2 teaspoons apple cider vinegar
- 1 tablespoon fresh parsley, chopped
- 1 tablespoon fresh basil, chopped
- 1 teaspoon celery seed
- 1 tablespoon Dijon mustard
- 1 tablespoon lemon juice
- 2 tablespoons olive oil
- ½ teaspoon sea salt
- ½ teaspoon black pepper

Preparation: 35 minutes | Cooking: 10 minutes | Servings: 8

Directions:

1. Preheat grill to medium-high, and spray with non-stick cooking spray.
2. Place potatoes on griddle and cook until tender, about 10 minutes.
3. Remove potatoes from grill and allow to cool for 10 minutes.

4. Combine dressing ingredients in a large mixing bowl and whisk until well-combined.

5. Fold in the potatoes until mixed well, and serve at room temperature or well-chilled from the refrigerator overnight.

Nutrition: Calories 132, Sodium 246 mg, Dietary Fiber 1.3 g, Fat 8.9 g, Carbohydrates 13.7 g, Protein 1.9 g

Baby Gem Lettuce with Balsamic & Goat Cheese

Ingredients:

- 4 Baby Gem lettuce heads, ends trimmed and quartered
- 3 tablespoon olive oil
- 1 teaspoon sea salt
- 1 teaspoon black pepper
- 3 stalks green onions
- 1 package soft goat's cheese, crumbled
- Balsamic glaze, for serving

Preparation: 10 minutes | Cook time: 10 minutes | Servings: 3

Directions:

1. Preheat the griddle to high heat.
2. Lay cut lettuce and green onion stalks on a baking sheet and coat with olive oil; salt and pepper each evenly.
3. Griddle the vegetables for 1 min per side or until slightly charred. Remove to a plate.
4. Drizzle with balsamic glaze and sprinkle with goat's cheese.
5. Serve warm with your favorite meal!

Nutrition: Calories 298, Sodium 751 mg, Dietary Fiber 5.8 g, Fat 20.1 g, Carbohydrates 28.9 g, Protein 6.2 g

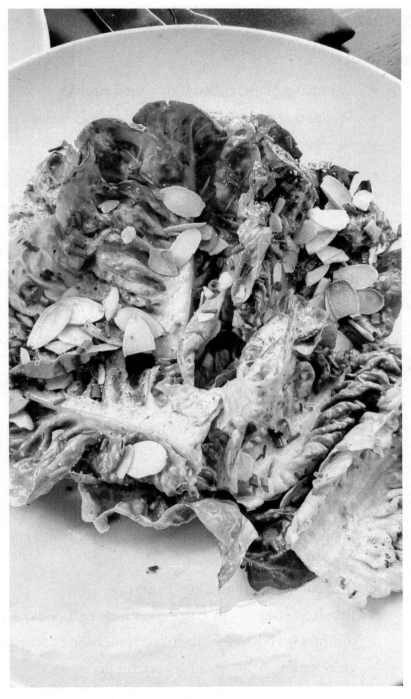

Balsamic Glazed Veggie Kabobs

Ingredients:

- ½ cup eggplant, cubed into 1-inch chunks
- ½ cup bell peppers, cubed into 1-inch chunks
- ½ cup zucchini, cubed into 1-inch chunks
- ½ cup red onion, cubed into 1-inch chunks
- 3 tablespoons olive oil
- 1 teaspoon garlic powder
- 1 teaspoon sea salt
- 1 teaspoon black pepper
- 1/4 cup balsamic glaze

Preparation: 10 minutes | Cooking: 8 minutes | Servings: 4 to 6

Directions:

1. Preheat griddle to medium-high heat.
2. Arrange vegetables on metal skewers in an alternating pattern.
3. Place on a baking sheet or piece of aluminum foil.
4. Whisk together the olive oil, garlic powder, salt, and pepper in a small mixing bowl and pour over skewers; turn skewers to coat well.
5. Preheat a grill to medium heat.
6. Brush skewers with balsamic glaze and cook 4 to 5 minutes on both sides until charred; basting with extra glaze often until vegetables are tender.

7. Remove kabobs to a serving tray and enjoy!

Nutrition: Calories 73, Sodium 314 mg, Dietary Fiber 0.9 g, Fat 7.1 g, Carbohydrates 3.1 g, Protein 0.5 g

Romaine Salad with Bacon & Blue Cheese

Ingredients:

- 3 romaine hearts
- 12 pieces of thick cut bacon
- 5 oz blue cheese crumbles

For the dressing:

- ¼ cup balsamic vinegar
- ¼ cup light olive oil
- ¼ teaspoon dried thyme
- ¼ teaspoon dried parsley
- ½ teaspoon dried oregano
- A little salt and pepper
- ¼ teaspoon Dijon mustard

Directions:

1. Preheat the griddle to medium-high heat on one side and high heat on the other
2. Lay the bacon on the medium-high side and griddle for 5 to 8 minutes on each side.
3. Slice each romaine heart in half and set aside.
4. Use a brush to collect a little bit of bacon grease, and brush onto the flat side of each Romaine half.
5. Place the romaine halves flat side down on the high heat side of the grill for 30 seconds each.

6. Remove the bacon to a paper towel lined plate, and chop into crumbles when cool.

7. Remove romaine halves to another plate.

8. Whisk the dressing ingredients together in a small mixing bowl and drizzle over romaine.

9. Top each romaine half with bacon and blue cheese crumbles to serve.

Nutrition: Calories 283, Sodium 866 mg, Dietary Fiber 0.6 g, Fat 25.1 g, Carbohydrates 2.9 g, Protein 12.7 g

Potato Salad with Bacon Vinaigrette

Ingredients:

For the potatoes:

- 7 medium red potatoes, quartered
- 1 sweet potato, peeled and cut into large chunks
- 1/4 cup mayonnaise
- 1 tablespoon Dijon mustard
- 2 teaspoons onion powder
- 2 teaspoons garlic powder
- 1/4 teaspoon celery seed
- Sea salt, to taste
- Freshly ground black pepper, to taste

For the vinaigrette:

- 2 slices bacon, cooked and chopped
- 1/4 cup extra-virgin olive oil
- 2 tablespoons red wine vinegar
- 2 shallots, minced
- 2 tablespoons fresh parsley, chopped

Preparation: 20 minutes | Cooking: 40 minutes | Servings: 4

Directions:

1. Preheat a griddle to medium.
2. Put the red potatoes in a large saucepan and cover with cold water by 2 inches. Bring the water to a boil over

high heat; after about 10 minutes, add the sweet potatoes.

3. Return to a boil and cook 10 additional minutes.
4. Drain the potatoes and set aside to cool.
5. Whisk the mayonnaise, mustard, onion powder, garlic powder, celery seed, salt and black pepper in medium mixing bowl.
6. Fold the cooled potatoes into the mayonnaise mixture.
7. Mix the vinaigrette ingredients together in a small bowl until well-combined.
8. Use tongs to place the potato pieces back on the hot grill and cook on all sides long enough to cook through and make grill marks, about 1 to 2 minutes per side: be sure to handle the potatoes gently so they don't fall apart.
9. Remove the potatoes from the grill and place in the bowl with the vinaigrette.
10. **Gently toss to coat completely and serve warm or cold.**

Nutrition: Calories 521, Sodium 521 mg, Dietary Fiber 7.7 g, Fat 22.3 g, Carbohydrates 72.1 g, Protein 12 g

Artichokes with Harissa-Honey Dip

Ingredients:

- 4 medium artichokes
- 1 lemon, juiced
- 4 tablespoons olive oil
- For the Harissa Dip:
- 1/2 cup mayonnaise
- 1 tablespoon harissa
- 1 tablespoon honey
- 1/4 teaspoon fresh ground pepper
- ¼ teaspoon sea salt

Preparation: 10 minutes | Cooking: 30 minutes | Servings: 4

Directions:

1. Cut a 1/2 inch off the top of each artichoke, then cut each in half vertically.
2. Trim the pointy ends off the leaves with scissors.
3. Cut out the fuzzy choke in the center of each and discard.
4. Fill a large pot with water and fit with a steaming rack. Place artichokes on rack and steam until they are tender and easily pierced with a fork, about 30 minutes.
5. Set aside to cool for 15 minutes.
6. Preheat grill to high heat.

7. Combine Harissa Dip ingredients in a small mixing bowl until well-combined and set aside.
8. Add lemon and oil to a large mixing bowl, and toss artichokes in lemon and oil.
9. Grill artichokes, cut side down, until nicely charred, about 4 to 5 minutes.
10. **Serve hot with harissa dip.**

Nutrition: Calories 328, Sodium 492 mg, Dietary Fiber 7.4 g, Fat 24.7 g, Carbohydrates 27.7 g, Protein: 4.9 g

Cumin Chili Potato Wedges

Ingredients:

- 3 large russet potatoes, scrubbed and cut into 1-inch thick wedges
- 1/3 cup olive oil
- 1 teaspoon cumin
- 1 teaspoon chili powder
- 1 teaspoon garlic powder
- 1 teaspoon kosher salt
- 1 teaspoon freshly ground black pepper

Preparation: 5 minutes | Cooking: 20 minutes | Servings: 3 to 4

Directions:

1. Mix together the cumin, chili powder, garlic powder, salt, and pepper in a small bowl and set aside.
2. Preheat one side of the grill to medium-high heat and the other on medium heat.
3. Brush the potatoes all over with olive oil and place over the hot side of the grill and cook until browned and crisp on both sides, about 2 to 3 minutes per side.
4. Move the potatoes to the cooler side of the grill, tent with foil, and continue to grill until cooked through, about 5 to 10 minutes longer.
5. Remove the potatoes from the grill to a large bowl.

6. Sprinkle with the spice mixture and toss to coat. Serve warm and enjoy.

Nutrition: Calories 343, Sodium 606 mg, Dietary Fiber 7.1 g, Fat 17.3 g, Carbohydrates 44.9 g, Protein 5 g

Chili Con Carne

Ingredients:

- Spice packet
- 1 teaspoon salt
- ½ teaspoon freshly ground black pepper
- 2 ½ teaspoons ground cumin
- 1 ½ teaspoon chili powder
- 1 teaspoon crushed chilies
- 1 tablespoon paprika
- 1 tablespoon dried oregano
- 1 cinnamon stick
- 1 bay leaf
- 1 ½ pounds lean ground beef
- 1 large onion, chopped
- 3 cloves garlic, chopped
- 2 (14.5-ounce) cans diced tomatoes with liquid
- 1 (15-ounce) can red kidney beans, rinsed and drained
- 1 (15-ounce) can black beans, rinsed and drained

Preparation: 10 minutes | Cooking: 1 hour and 10 minutes | Servings: 6

Directions:

1. At home, combine the necessary spices in a lidded container or resealable bag.

2. At the campsite, place your 12-inch Dutch oven over 18 briquettes.
3. Sauté the ground beef until it is browned and drain any excess grease.
4. Add the onion and cook until it is tender, then stir in the garlic. Add the spices and tomatoes.
5. Cover the pot, and arrange it with 16 briquettes underneath and 8 on top. Cook for 45 minutes, maintaining a temperature around 325°F.
6. Add the beans and cook for 15 more minutes. Remove the cinnamon stick and bay leaf before serving.

Nutrition: Calories 318, Fat 12.4 g, Carbohydrates 30.1 g, Sugar 7.5 g, Protein 19.4g, Sodium 1020 mg

Hodge Podge

Ingredients:

- 1 ½ cups fresh green beans, trimmed and snapped
- 1 ½ cups fresh wax beans, trimmed and snapped
- 1 ½ cups diced carrot
- 2 cups cubed new potatoes
- ½ teaspoon salt
- ¼ cup salted butter
- ¼ cup heavy cream
- 1 tablespoon all-purpose flour

- 1 cup whole milk
- Salt and pepper to taste

Preparation: 10 minutes | Cooking 45 minutes | Servings: 6

<u>Directions:</u>

1. Place the beans, carrots, potatoes, and salt in a saucepan and add just enough water to cover.
2. Simmer for 30–40 minutes, until all the vegetables are tender.
3. Stir in the butter and cream.
4. Whisk the flour into the milk and add it to the pot. Cook until thickened and season with salt and pepper to taste.

Nutrition: Calories 199, Fat 12.8 g, Carbohydrates: 18.5 g, Protein 3.9 g, Sodium 301.5 mg

Campfire Chicken and Dumplings

Ingredients

- 1 whole fryer chicken, 4-5 pounds
- 4 stalks celery, sliced
- 1 large onion, diced
- 2 medium carrots, peeled and sliced
- 1 teaspoon salt
- 1 teaspoon black pepper
- 2 teaspoons garlic powder
- 1 (14.5-ounce) can low-Sodium chicken broth

For the dumplings

- 1 ½ cups white whole wheat flour
- ½ teaspoon salt
- 5 tablespoons butter
- 1 egg
- ½ cup milk
- 1 tablespoon dried parsley

Preparation: 10 minutes | Cooking: 45 minutes | Servings: 6

Directions:

1. Place a large Dutch oven over 18–20 briquettes. Add the chicken with enough water to just cover. Put in the celery, onion, carrots, salt, black pepper, and broth.
2. Bring the pot to a boil and then transfer it to less intense heat. Keep it simmering for an hour.

3. Meanwhile, prepare the dumpling batter. Combine the flour and salt and cut in the butter. Mix in the egg, milk, parsley, and pepper, and knead for about 5 minutes.

4. Carefully remove the chicken to a strainer and let it cool a little. Remove and discard any skin and Fat, and pull the meat from the bones.

5. Skim the fat from the broth and add the cooked chicken back in. Taste the broth and add more seasonings if desired.

6. Pull off little bits of the dumpling dough and roll them into balls if desired. Drop them into the broth.

7. Cover the pot and bring it to a simmer. Cook, covered, for 20 minutes.

Nutrition: Calories 463, Fat 16.3 g, Carbohydrates 25.2 g, Sugar 3.4 g, Protein 50.1g, Sodium 940.6 mg

Tomato Chickpea Soup

Ingredients:

- ¼ cup extra-virgin olive oil
- 2 medium yellow onions, diced
- 1 stalk celery, diced
- 4 cloves garlic, minced
- 1 bunch kale, trimmed and chopped (about 3 cups)
- 2 (28-ounce) cans crushed tomatoes
- 1 quart low-Sodium vegetable stock
- 1 cup basmati rice, rinsed
- ¼ cup tomato paste
- 2 (15-ounce) cans chickpeas, drained and rinsed
- 1 teaspoon salt
- ½ teaspoon black pepper
- Hot sauce or crushed chilies, to taste

Preparation: 10 minutes | Cooking: 30 minutes | Servings: 8

Directions:

1. In your Dutch oven over 18 coals, warm the oil and sauté the onion and celery for 3–5 minutes. Stir in the garlic and cook until fragrant.
2. Add the kale, and stir a minute or two until it begins to wilt.

3. Add the tomatoes, vegetable stock, and rice. Bring the mixture to a boil and let it simmer for 15–20 minutes.

4. Add the tomato paste, chickpeas, salt, pepper, and hot sauce. Cook to heat through, and serve.

Nutrition: Calories 323, Fat 9.3 g, Carbohydrates 52.9 g, Sugar 16.8 g, Protein 11.6g, Sodium 812.8 mg

Spiced Lentil Soup

Ingredients:

- Spice packet
- 2 teaspoons ground turmeric
- 1 ½ teaspoons ground cumin
- ¼ teaspoon cinnamon
- ½ teaspoon sea salt
- ½ teaspoon black pepper
- Pinch red pepper flakes
- 2 tablespoons extra virgin olive oil
- 1 large onion, diced
- 3 cloves garlic, minced
- ¾ cup red lentils, rinsed and drained
- 1 (15-ounce) can diced tomatoes, with juices
- 1 (15-ounce) can light coconut milk
- 1 quart low-Sodium vegetable broth
- 3 cups packed baby spinach
- 1 tablespoon fresh lemon juice

Preparation: 5 minutes | Cooking: 30 minutes | Servings: 4

Directions:

1. At home, combine the spices in a small, lidded container, and seal.

2. In your Dutch oven over 18 coals, warm the oil and sauté the onion and garlic until tender.

3. Add the spices and the lentils and mix well. Continue cooking for another minute or two, but don't let the spices burn.

4. Add the tomatoes, coconut milk, and broth. Bring it to a boil and simmer, uncovered, for 20 minutes, or until the lentils are tender.

5. Add the spinach and lemon juice, and cook until the spinach wilts.

Nutrition: Calories 254, Fat 14.9 g, Carbohydrates 25.4 g, Sugar 4.8 g, Protein 7.3 g, Sodium 744.3 mg

Chicken Stew Recipe

Ingredients:

- 1 broiler/fryer chicken (3 ½ to 4 pounds), cut up
- 3 to 4 medium potatoes, peeled and sliced
- 1 cup thinly sliced carrots
- 1 medium green pepper, sliced
- 1 can (10-3/4 ounces) condensed cream of mushroom soup, undiluted
- 1/4 cup water
- 1/2 teaspoon salt
- 1/4 teaspoon pepper

Preparation: 10 minutes | Cooking: 20 to 25 minutes | Servings: 4

Directions:

1. Grill chicken, covered, over medium heat for three minutes on all sides.
2. Place 2 items of chicken on every of 4 double thicknesses of professional quality foil (about eighteen in. x 12 in.).
3. Divide the potatoes, carrots, and sweet pepper among the packets.
4. Fold foil around mixture and seal tightly.
5. Grill, covered, over medium heat for 20-25 minutes on all sides or till chicken juices run clear.

6. Open foil rigorously to permit steam to flee.

Nutrition: Calories 36, Fat 2.1 g, Carbohydrates 2.5 g, Sugar 1.9 g, Protein 1.8 g, Sodium 333.5 mg

Barbeque Stew Packet

Ingredients:

- 4 medium potatoes, diced
- 1 large onion, slivered
- 8 sliced carrots
- 1-pound stew meat
- 1 can cream of mushroom soup
- Salt and pepper

Preparation: 10 minutes | Cooking: 25 to 30 minutes | Servings: 4

Directions:

1. Mix all at once in an exceedingly giant bowl, give out into four servings and wrap in foil packets.
2. Grill over medium heat until done, 25-30 minutes, turning halfway through cookery time.

Nutrition: Calories 25, Fat 1.8 g, Carbohydrates 2.3 g, Sugar 2.0 g, Protein 1.2 g, Sodium 309.7 mg

Tin Foil Stew

Ingredients:

- Heavy duty aluminum foil
- 6 oz. blade roast, trimmed and cut into 1 inch cubes
- 1 potato, cubed
- 2 carrots, sliced
- 1 onion, chopped
- 1 clove crushed garlic
- 1 pinch salt
- 1 pinch ground black pepper
- 1 tbsp butter 1 tbsp. water

Preparation: 10 minutes | Cooking: 1 hour | Servings: 4

Directions:

1. On a large square sheet of foil, layer beef, potato cubes, carrots, onion and garlic.
2. Sprinkle with salt and pepper, top with butter and a tbsp of water.
3. Form a foil packet.
4. Grill on high for about 1 hour.
5. Serve with your camping buddies and enjoy!

Nutrition: Calories 392.7, Total Fat 18.1 g, Saturated Fat 7.2 g, Cholesterol 63.8 mg, Sodium 91.9 mg, Potassium 1,203.1 mg, Total Carbohydrate 38.0 g, Dietary Fiber 4.7 g, Protein 19.5 g

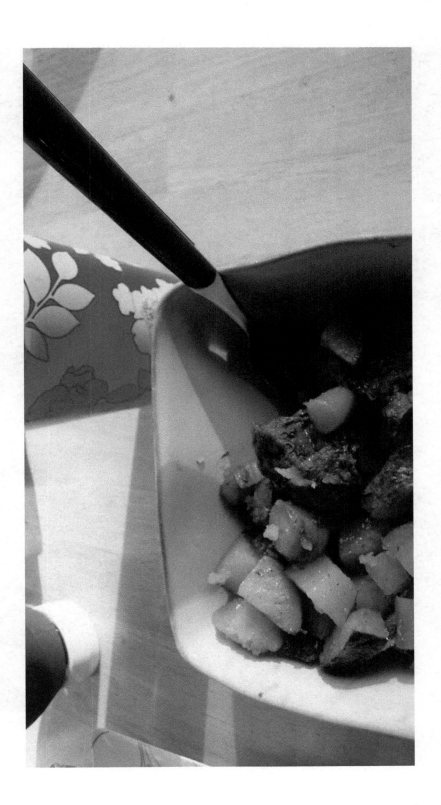

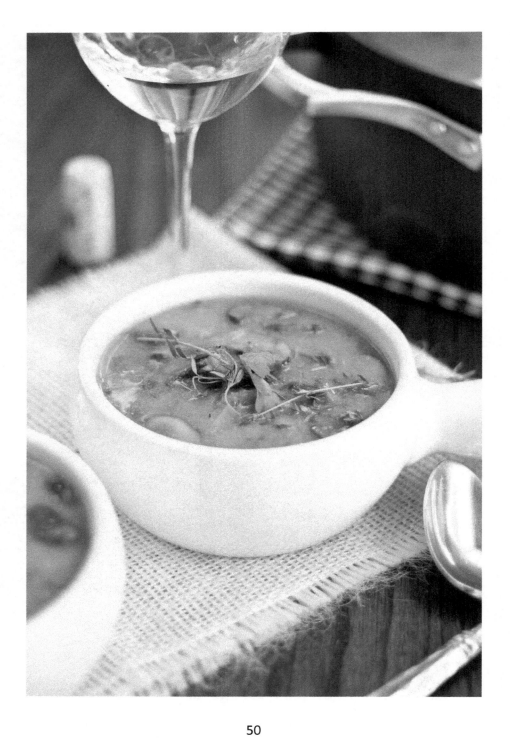

Wild Rice Soup

Ingredients:

- Dried potatoes, 1 cup
- Leek soup, 3 packages
- Wild rice, 1 cup, uncooked
- Salt, to taste
- Pepper, to taste
- Powdered milk, 1 cup
- Cheddar cheese, 1 chunk

Preparation: 10 minutes | Cooking: 25 minutes | Servings: 8

Directions:

1. Reconstitute potatoes and rice separately in a zip top plastic bag all day.
2. Simmer potatoes in water until fork tender then add leek soup mix, powdered milk and 4 cups water.
3. Boil the soup and add rice.
4. Season with salt and pepper.
5. Chop cheese into small pieces and add to the soup.
6. Add 2 cups water and cook until the cheese has melted and the soup has a slightly thick consistency.

Nutrition: Calories 170.6, Total Fat 3.8 g, Saturated Fat 1.4 g, Cholesterol 48.2 mg, Sodium 1,371.6 mg, Potassium 546.1 mg, Total Carbohydrate 15.9 g, Dietary Fiber 1.1 g, Protein 17.3 g

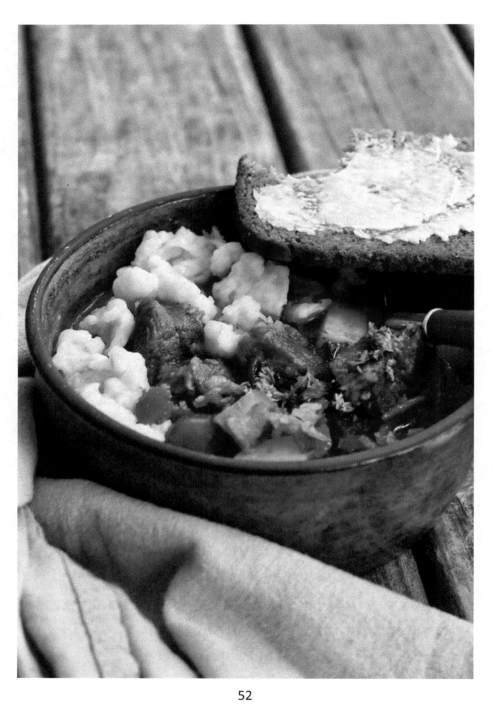

Fast Goulash

Ingredients:

- 3 Tbsp oil and butter
- 2 cloves garlic (or 1/2 teaspoon powdered garlic)
- 1 large onion
- 1-pound(s) ground beef
- 1 (26-ounce) can of whole tomatoes
- 1/2 tsp dill seed
- 1 tsp parsley
- salt and pepper to taste

Preparation: 5 minutes | Cooking: 30 minutes | Servings: 4

Directions:

1. In 3 tbsp of oil or butter, sauté 2 cloves of fresh garlic, peeled and chopped (or later, when browning the meat, add 1/2 to 1 tsp of powdered garlic, depending on your taste.

2. While the garlic is simmering, peel and slice (about 1/4' thick slices) 1 large onion (of any kind). Do not chop.

3. Add it in its whole rings, and turn up the heat all the way.

4. When the onions are soft and beginning to brown, add 1 lb of ground beef, not too lean as Fat adds flavor.

5. Mix with the onion and garlic and cook until brown. Add salt and pepper to taste. While the meat is browning, open a 26 oz can of whole tomatoes.

6. When the meat is brown, add the juice from the can and the tomatoes, tearing them into small pieces with your fingers.

7. This creates a juice, rather than a gravy. If the tomatoes come in a thick sauce, add water until it becomes juice-like. Add 1/2 tsp of dill seed and 1 tsp of dried (or fresh, chopped) parsley. Cover and simmer.

8. Cook 1 cup or your favorite rice.

9. When the rice is done, so is the goulash. Place 1/2 cup of rice on each plate and cover with goulash, making sure to serve with plenty of juice.

Nutrition: Calories 170, Sodium 556 mg, Dietary Fiber 0.8 g, Fat 9.9 g, Carbohydrates 5.9 g, Protein 3.9 g

A Mean Three-Bean Salad

Ingredients:

- 2 15 oz. cans pinto beans
- 2 15 oz. cans kidney beans
- 2 15 oz. cans garbanzo beans
- 1 c red onion, thinly sliced
- 1 c green bell pepper, chopped
- 1 c red bell pepper, chopped
- 1/2 c celery
- 3/4 c red wine vinegar
- 1/2 c sugar
- 1/2 c olive oil
- 1/2 tsp dry mustard
- 1/2 tsp salt
- 2 Tbsp parsley, chopped
- 1 Tbsp fresh cilantro, chopped
- 1 tsp fresh oregano, chopped

Preparation: 10 minutes | Cooking: None | Servings: 4

Directions:

1. Drain all the beans; put into a large mixing bowl.
2. Add red onion, bell peppers, and celery.
3. In a small bowl, combine vinegar, sugar, olive oil, salt, mustard, cilantro, parsley, and oregano.

4. Pour over beans and veggies; toss to mix well.

5. Cover and refrigerate several hours or overnight, stirring occasionally.

Nutrition: Calories 166, Sodium 466 mg, Dietary Fiber 2.5 g, Fat 14.2 g, Carbohydrates 7.5 g, Protein 4.2 g

Mashed Potatoes

Ingredients:

- 8 mashed potatoes
- 4 strips bacon, diced
- 2 medium onions, thinly sliced
- 1 Parmesan cheese, freshly grated
- 3 cloves garlic, minced
- 2 Tbsp fresh parsley, chopped
- 1 stick butter
- Salt and pepper to taste

Preparation: 5 minutes | Cooking: 10 minutes | Servings: 12

Directions:

1. Peel and boil potatoes; drain.
2. Fry bacon until crisp; add onion and cook for five minutes, adding garlic near the end.
3. Add bacon mixture and butter to potatoes, mixing thoroughly.
4. Add seasonings as desired.

Nutrition: Calories 126, Sodium 63 mg, Dietary Fiber 2.9 g, Fat 7.2 g, Carbohydrates 13.9 g, Protein 3 g

All Fruit Salad

Ingredients:

- Watermelon
- Cantelope
- Green or red grapes
- Apples
- Pineapple
- Strawberries
- Blueberries
- Raspberries
- Oranges
- Grapefruit

Preparation: 10 minutes | Cooking: None | Servings: 6 to 8

Directions:

1. Mix all fruit together - sweeten with sugar if you want and then top fruit with bananas around the edge and in the center.
2. Serve in bowls, and top with whipped crème and a cherry.

Nutrition: Calories 206, Sodium 812 mg, Dietary Fiber 2.9 g, Fat 15.8 g, Carbohydrates 11.2 g, Protein 7 g

All in One Burger and Sides

Ingredients:

- Hamburger
- Potatoes
- Corn on the Cob

Preparation: 10 minutes | Cooking: 30 to 45 minutes | Servings: 2

Directions:

1. Make a hamburger patty with your seasoning.
2. Cut a potato slice about 2" thick.
3. Put a corn on the cob, one that is about 4" long.
4. Wrap all this in aluminum foil and seal.
5. Cook this on the grill about 30 minutes to 45 minutes.
6. You have a complete meal in one wrap.

Nutrition: Calories 148, Sodium 503 mg, Dietary Fiber 3.8 g, Fat 8 g, Carbohydrates 16.8 g, Protein 3.9 g

Amarillo Steak

Ingredients:

- 2 - 2.5 pound(s) lean beef: Top Round, Flank steak or London Broil
- 1/3 c virgin olive oil
- 1/3 c reconstituted lemon juice or juice of one lemon
- 2 cloves garlic, crushed or equivalent dried
- 1/4 tsp salt
- 1/4 tsp pepper

Preparation: 10 minutes | Cooking: 20 minutes | Servings: 6

Directions:

1. Combine marinade ingredients in a Ziploc freezer bag and add steak. Refrigerate 6-8 hours.
2. Remove steak and discard marinade.
3. Grill steak over medium heat about 10 minutes per side or to desired doneness. For medium doneness, that's about 150 degrees.
4. Transfer steak to cutting board and allow to sit for 10 minutes. Slice diagonally across the grain into thin strips.
5. Great with a cold potato salad on a summer day! Refrigerated leftover strips are wonderful on a sandwich or salad the next day.

Nutrition: Calories 81, Sodium 56 mg, Dietary Fiber 0.9 g, Fat 4.9 g, Carbohydrates 3.8 g, Protein 5.7 g

Antipasta Dip

Ingredients:

- 2 large tomatoes (finely chopped)
- 1 small can chop green chilis
- 1 small can chop black olives
- 3 Tbsp olive oil
- 3 or 4 green onions (chopped)
- 1 1/2 Tbsp vinegar
- 1 green pepper (finely chopped)
- 1 small jar chopped pimento
- 1 Tbsp garlic salt

Preparation: 10 minutes | Cooking: None | Servings: 8

Directions:

1. Mix all ingredients together and marinate in refrigerator for a while.
2. Serve as dip with nacho chips

Nutrition: Calories 108, Sodium 65 mg, Dietary Fiber 2.1 g, Fat 5.2 g, Carbohydrates 9.4 g, Protein 7.3 g

Arkansas Potatoes

Ingredients

- 1 package fully cooked smoked sausage, sliced
- 1 large onion
- Several small red/yellow potatoes
- Salt and pepper
- Seasoning salt

Preparation: 5 minutes | Cooking: 20 minutes | Servings: 2

Directions:

1. Slice onion, potatoes, and place in fireproof skillet.
2. Add water to keep from scorching.
3. Add seasonings to taste along with smoked sausage.
4. Cook for 20 minutes.

Nutrition: Calories 151, Sodium 174 mg, Dietary Fiber 1 g, Fat 7.7 g, Carbohydrates 4.8 g, Protein 14.7 g

Asian Marinade

Ingredients:

- 1/4 soy sauce
- 3 Tbsp honey
- 2 Tbsp vinegar
- 3/4 olive oil
- 2 green onions, finely chopped
- 1 1/2 tsp garlic powder
- 1 1/2 tsp ground ginger

Preparation: 5 minutes | Cooking: None | Servings: 2

Directions:

1. Wisk together all ingredients in a medium sized bowl, and pour into a zip lock bag or airtight container.
2. This recipe marinates up to 2 pounds of meat.

Nutrition: Calories 338, Sodium 333 mg, Dietary Fiber 4.1 g, Fat 12.9 g, Carbohydrates 20.3 g, Protein 34.9 g

Apricot Pork Chops

Ingredients:

- 1 pork chop
- 1 cup apricot preserves
- 1 tablespoon butter, melted
- 1 teaspoon balsamic vinegar

Preparation: 5 minutes | Cooking: 15 to 20 minutes | Servings: 1

Directions:

1. **Combine butter, apricot preserves, and vinegar and stir together.**
2. Place pork chop on foil and coat with peach preserve mixture.
3. Wrap tightly in a foil packet.
4. **Cook for 15 to 20 minutes, or until pork is cooked all the way through.**

Nutrition: Calories 82, Sodium 53 mg, Dietary Fiber 2.8 g, Fat 3.8 g, Carbohydrates 11.5 g, Protein 2.2 g.

Bacon Burgers

Ingredients:

- 1 hamburger patty
- 2 sliced of bacon
- 1 slice of cheddar cheese
- Salt and pepper, to taste
- Hamburger bun
- Condiments

Preparation: 10 minutes | Cooking: 12 to 15 minutes | Servings: 1

Directions:

1. **Wrap bacon pieces around hamburger and pin in place with a toothpick.**
2. **If you wrap the bacon around the top and place it under the hamburger, you can probably get away with not using a toothpick.**
3. Place on foil and wrap foil tightly around the burger.
4. Cook for 12 to 15 minutes, or until burger is cooked to your liking.
5. **Remove from heat and open carefully.**
6. Place cheese on bacon burger and place burger on bun.
7. Add condiments to your liking.

NOTE: These burgers can be made in advance and wrapped in foil. Cook the bacon burgers ahead of time and build the burgers at home. When you're hungry, all you'll have to do is warm up the burgers up until they're cooked all the way through, and the cheese is melted. We usually build 15 to 20 burgers in advance, so the kids can warm one up as a snack anytime they want.

Nutrition: Calories 215, Sodium 99 mg, Dietary Fiber 8.9 g, Fat 5.8 g, Carbohydrates 35.9 g, Protein 8.9 g

Burger and Beans

Ingredients:

- ¼ pound hamburger
- ½ onion, diced
- ½ cup baked beans
- ¼ cup barbecue sauce
- A handful of bread crumbs
- Salt and pepper, to taste

Preparation: 10 minutes | Cooking: 20 to 25 minutes | Servings: 1

Directions:

1. **Combine the hamburger, onion, barbecue sauce and breadcrumbs, salt and pepper in a bowl and mix together.**
2. Form the hamburger into a patty and place the patty on the foil.
3. Pour beans over the top.
4. **Seal the foil packet tightly.**
5. Cook for 20 to 25 minutes, or until hamburger is cooked to your liking.

Nutrition: Calories 246, Sodium 513 mg, Dietary Fiber 1.3 g, Fat 12.8 g, Carbohydrates 7.2 g, Protein 19.3 g

Chuck Steak Stew

Ingredients:

- 1-pound chuck steak, cubed
- 1 package onion soup mix
- 2 potatoes, peeled and cut into chunks
- 2 carrots, peeled and cut into coins
- ¼ cup water
- ½ cup mushrooms, sliced
- 2 tablespoons olive oil
- Salt and pepper, to taste

Preparation: 10 minutes | Cooking: 30 to 45 minutes | Servings: 4

Directions:

1. **Add all ingredients to a foil packet and mix together.**
2. **Wrap packet up.**
3. **Leave room for steam to form.**
4. **Cook packet for 30 to 45 minutes, or until steak is cooked all the way through and the vegetables are soft.**
5. **If you want a thicker stew, add a few tablespoons of flour at a time and stir it in until the stew is of the desired consistency.**

Nutrition: Calories 249, Sodium 792 mg, Dietary Fiber 0.7 g, Fat 20.1 g, Carbohydrates 4.2 g, Protein 13.3 g

Cowboy Steak Packets

Ingredients:

- ½ pound sirloin steak, cubed
- ½ cup broccoli florets
- 1 red bell pepper, seeded and sliced
- 1 small onion, sliced
- 4 new potatoes, sliced
- 2 tablespoons fresh parsley
- 1 tablespoon garlic pepper
- 2 tablespoons olive oil
- Salt and pepper, to taste

Preparation: 10 minutes | Cooking: 20 to 25 minutes | Servings: 4

Directions:

1. **Add all ingredients to a bowl and mix together.**
2. Place contents of bowl into a foil packet and seal it tight.
3. Place in campfire and cook for 20 to 25 minutes, or until steak and veggies are cooked to your liking.

Nutrition: Calories 159, Sodium 573 mg, Dietary Fiber 1 g, Fat 14.1 g, Carbohydrates 4.8 g, Protein 4.9 g

Ham, Asparagus and Potatoes

Ingredients:

- 1 large ham steak, cut into pieces
- 10 asparagus spears, broken into pieces
- 4 small red potatoes, cut into pieces
- ½ cup Alfredo sauce

Directions:

1. **Combine all ingredients in a foil packet.**
2. Seal the foil packet, leaving room for steam.
3. Cook for 15 to 20 minutes, or until asparagus is soft.

Nutrition: Calories 616, Sodium 1349 mg, Dietary Fiber 5.1 g, Fat 34.7 g, Carbohydrates 56.8 g, Protein 11 g.

Ham and Pineapple

Ingredients:

- 1 ham steak, cut into chunks
- 3 pineapple rings, cut into chunks
- 1 sweet potato, cubed
- 2 tablespoons brown sugar
- 2 tablespoons butter

Preparation: 30 minutes | Cooking: 15 to 20 minutes | Servings: 4

Directions:

1. **Add all ingredients to foil packet.**
2. Seal packet up, leaving room for steam.
3. Cook for 15 to 20 minutes or until pineapple and potatoes are cooked.
4. **Flip packet after 10 minutes.**
5. Let cool for 10 minutes before opening packet.

Nutrition: Calories 539, Sodium 852 mg, Dietary Fiber 6.4 g, Fat 35.3 g, Carbohydrates 47.2 g, Protein 6.9 g

Ham and Swiss

Ingredients:

- Ham lunch meat, thinly sliced
- ½ loaf sourdough bread
- 2 tablespoons butter
- 5 slices of Swiss cheese

Preparation: 10 minutes | Cooking: 15 to 20 minutes | Servings: 5

Directions:

1. **Slice the loaf of sourdough bread into 10 slices and place the loaf on the foil.**
2. Spread a bit of butter between every other piece.
3. Place a slice of Swiss cheese and few pieces of lunchmeat next to the same pieces of bread you spread the butter on, making 5 sandwiches.
4. **Wrap the loaf of bread up tightly.**
5. Cook for 15 to 20 minutes, or until the cheese is melted all the way through. Flip the foil packet after 7 minutes.

Nutrition: Calories 68, Sodium 1554 mg, Dietary Fiber 0.6 g, Fat 2.5 g, Carbohydrates 3.5 g, Protein 7.3 g

Hamburger and Veggies

Ingredients:

- ½ pound ground beef
- ½ can cream of mushroom soup
- ¼ cup sliced mushrooms
- ¼ cup carrot coins
- ¼ cup corn niblets
- Salt and pepper, to taste

Preparation: 5 minutes | Cooking: 30 to 45 minutes | Servings: 4

Directions:

1. **Add all ingredients to a foil packet and seal the packet up.**
2. Cook for 30 to 45 minutes, or until veggies are soft and hamburger is cooked.

Nutrition: Calories 118, Sodium 208 mg, Dietary Fiber 2.6 g, Fat 5.4 g, Carbohydrates 16.4 g, Protein 7.6 g

Oriental Chicken

Ingredients:

- 4 chicken breasts, boneless and skinless
- 1/2 cup sweet and sour sauce
- 1 can pineapple chunks, 8 oz., drained
- 1/2 bell pepper, cut into thin strips
- 1/4 onion, cut into wedges
- 1/2 cup chow mein noodles
- Heavy duty aluminum foil – 4 pieces 18" x 18"

Preparation: 20 minutes | Cooking: 30 to 40 minutes | Servings: 4

Directions:

1. Spray each piece foil with non-stick cooking spray.
2. Place one chicken breast in the center of each foil and top with one tablespoon of sweet and sour sauce and 1/4 of the pineapple chunks.
3. Add 1/4 of pepper strips and onion wedges.
4. Top off with remaining sweet and sour sauce.
5. Fold foil loosely over veggies and chicken to form a tent packet, folding and crimping seams tightly.
6. Rotate packets 1/2 turn every 10 minutes on the grill.
7. When done, place a portion of chow mein noodles on top of the ingredients in each packet and serve.

8. Place foil packet on hot coals or a campfire grill for 30 to 40 minutes. Or place foil packet in covered grill on medium-low heat for 15 to 22 minutes.

Nutrition: Calories 151, Sodium 1338 mg, Dietary Fiber 1.7 g, Fat 9.7 g, Carbohydrates 8.9 g, Protein 9.8 g

Spicy Jerk Wings

Ingredients:

- 6 chicken wings, split
- 4 tablespoons jerk seasoning
- 2 tablespoons vegetable oil
- 1/4 cup cilantro, chopped
- 3 lemon wedges
- Heavy-duty aluminum foil - 18" x 24"

Preparation: 15 minutes | Cooking: 25 minutes | Servings: 6

Directions:

1. Combine jerk seasoning and oil and coat chicken with mixture.
2. Spray foil with non-stick cooking spray.
3. Place the wings in the center of foil and pour remaining mixture over them.
4. Fold the foil loosely to create a tent packet, folding and crimping seams tightly.
5. Place over hot coals, rotating 1/4 turn at half done.
6. When wings are cooked, sprinkle cilantro on them and serve with lemons.
7. Place foil packet on hot coals or a campfire grill for 25 minutes.
8. Or place foil packet in uncovered grill on medium heat for 25 minutes.

Nutrition: Calories 413, Sodium 1424 mg, Dietary Fiber 2.7 g, Fat 25.6 g, Carbohydrates 19.4 g, Protein 26 g

Chicken in the Garden

Ingredients:

- 4 chicken breasts, boneless and skinless
- 8 small potatoes (or 2 baking potatoes, peeled and cut in fourths)
- 8 small tomatoes
- 4 slices of onion
- 8 large mushroom slices
- 8 green pepper rings, sliced
- 4 teaspoons Worcestershire sauce
- Salt and pepper to taste
- 1/4 teaspoon paprika
- 4 tablespoons butter
- Heavy duty aluminum foil – 4 pieces of 18" x 24"

Preparation: 15 minutes | Cooking: 30 to 40 minutes | Servings: 4

Directions:

1. Cut each chicken breast into 2 pieces. Any pieces of chicken that are an inch thick or more, cut again. Spray foil with non-stick cooking spray. In each of the four pieces of foil, layer 2 cut up pieces of chicken, 2 potatoes, 2 tomatoes, 1 onion slice, 2 mushroom slices, 2 green pepper rings, 1 teaspoon Worcestershire

sauce, and sprinkle with salt, pepper and paprika. Dot with 1 tablespoon butter.

2. Fold the foil loosely to form a tent packet, folding and crimping seams tightly. Cook until chicken is opaque and potatoes are tender, rotating 1/2 turn at half done.

3. Place foil packets on hot coals or a campfire grill for 30 to 40 minutes.

4. Or place foil packets in covered grill on medium-low heat for 18 to 22 minutes.

Nutrition: Calories 158, Sodium 80 mg, Dietary Fiber 4.7 g, Fat 11.7 g, Carbohydrates 13.8 g, Protein 2.3 g

Lemon Barbecued Chicken

Ingredients:

- 3 chicken breasts, bone-in
- 3 tablespoons onion, chopped
- 3 tablespoons butter
- 3 tablespoons brown sugar
- 3/4 teaspoon dry mustard
- 3/4 teaspoon salt
- 3/4 teaspoon pepper
- 3 tablespoons lemon juice
- Heavy-duty aluminum foil – 3 pieces of 18" x 24"

Preparation: 15 minutes | Cooking: 30 to 45 minutes | Servings: 3

Directions:

1. Spray foil with non-stick cooking spray.
2. Lightly brown chicken in butter.
3. Center one piece of chicken on each piece of foil.
4. In the same skillet, sauté onions; sprinkle over chicken. Mix brown sugar, mustard, salt and pepper.
5. Sprinkle 1/3 of the brown sugar mixture on top of each chicken breast.
6. Rinse skillet with 3 tablespoons lemon juice and pour over chicken.

7. Fold the foil tightly to form a flat packet, crimping seams securely.

8. Cook using one of the options below. Place foil packet on hot coals or a campfire grill for 30 to 45 minutes. Or place foil packet in covered grill on medium-low heat for 22 to 25 minutes.

Nutrition: Calories 312, Sodium 345 mg, Dietary Fiber 17.7 g, Fat 7.4 g, Carbohydrates 43.2 g, Protein 20.1 g

Italian-Style Chicken

Ingredients:

- 2,5 to 3 lb. chicken, cut up, bone-in
- 4 small potatoes
- 2 medium zucchini
- 1/4 cup sliced pitted ripe olives
- 1 can tomato sauce, 8 oz.
- 2 teaspoons dried oregano, crushed
- 2 tablespoons butter or margarine
- Parmesan cheese, shredded
- Salt and pepper to taste
- Heavy-duty aluminum foil – 4 pieces 18" x 18"

Preparation: 15 minutes | Cooking: 45 to 60 minutes | Servings: 4

Directions:

1. Spray foil with non-stick cooking spray. Cut potatoes into 1/8-inch slices; divide onto 4 pieces of foil; sprinkle with salt and pepper. Cut zucchini into 1/4-inch slices; place on top of potatoes. Top with chicken pieces, olives, tomato sauce, oregano, and more salt and pepper. Dot with butter or margarine.

2. Fold the foil loosely to form a tent packet, folding and crimping seams tightly. Cook using one of the options

below. Add parmesan cheese to the top of ingredients in packet when done.

3. Place foil packet on hot coals or a campfire grill for 45 to 60 minutes, turning occasionally.

4. Or place foil packet in covered grill on medium-low heat for 30 to 35 minutes, turning occasionally.

Nutrition: Calories 350, Sodium 1032 mg, Dietary Fiber 1.3 g, Fat 35.3 g, Carbohydrates 7.9 g, Protein 3.8 g

Chicken with Mushrooms

Ingredients:

- 2 chicken breasts, split in half, bone-in
- 4 tablespoons butter
- 1/2 lb. fresh mushrooms, sliced or 1 can, 6 oz., drained
- 1/2 teaspoon rosemary
- 3/4 teaspoon salt
- 1/4 teaspoon pepper
- 4 tablespoons flour
- 1-pint light cream
- Heavy duty aluminum foil – 4 pieces of 18" x 24"

Preparation: 15 minutes | Cooking: 30 to 45 minutes | Servings: 4

Directions:

1. In a skillet, brown chicken breasts very lightly in butter. Spray foil with non-stick cooking spray. Place a chicken breast in center of each piece of foil. Sauté mushrooms quickly in same skillet and add 1/4 of mixture to each piece of foil; season with rosemary, 1/4 teaspoon salt, 1/4 teaspoon pepper. Add flour to butter remaining in skillet; stir and cook 2 minutes. Add cream, stir and cook until sauce is thickened. Add 1/2 teaspoon salt and a sprinkling of pepper. Pour over chicken breasts, dividing equally.

2. Fold the foil loosely to form a tent packet, folding and crimping seams tightly. Cook per instructions below.

3. Place foil packet on hot coals or a campfire grill for 30 to 45 minutes.

4. Or place foil packet in covered grill on medium-low heat for 22 to 25 minutes.

Nutrition: Calories 311, Sodium 802 mg, Dietary Fiber 9.5 g, Fat 9.7 g, Carbohydrates 39.6 g, Protein 18.2 g

Tropical Chicken

Ingredients:

- 3 chicken breasts, bone-in
- 3 slices pineapple, drained
- 1/2 cup slivered almonds
- 1/4 teaspoon rosemary
- 1/4 teaspoon tarragon
- Salt and pepper to taste
- Heavy duty aluminum foil – 3 pieces of 18" x 24"

Preparation: 15 minutes | Cooking: 30 to 45 minutes | Servings: 3

Directions:

1. Spray foil with non-stick cooking spray.
2. Brown chicken lightly in butter and place each chicken breast in the center of a piece of foil.
3. In same skillet, brown 3 slices of pineapple and 1/2 cup slivered almonds.
4. Divide evenly and arrange over each chicken breast.
5. Sprinkle each chicken with salt, pepper, rosemary, and tarragon – either fresh or dried.
6. Fold the foil tightly to form a flat packet, crimping seams securely.
7. Cook using one of the options below. Place foil packet on hot coals or a campfire grill for 30 to 45 minutes.

Or place foil packet in covered grill on medium-low heat for 22 to 25 minutes.

Nutrition: Calories 335, Sodium 600 mg, Dietary Fiber 22.2 g, Fat 7.2 g, Carbohydrates 47.6 g, Protein 21.4 g

Chicken Salad on a Bun

Ingredients:

- 2 cups chicken, chopped
- 6 green olives, chopped
- 2 tablespoons pickle relish
- 1/2 cup mayonnaise
- 2 hard-boiled eggs, chopped
- 2 tablespoons onion, chopped
- 1/4-pound American cheese, cubed in small pieces
- 12 small hamburger buns
- Heavy-duty aluminum foil – 12 pieces 18" x 12"

Preparation: 10 minutes | Cooking: 15 to 20 minutes | Servings: 6

Directions:

1. Mix all ingredients. Divide chicken mixture evenly between 12 buns.
2. Wrap each bun in foil, crimping seams tightly.
3. Place foil packet on hot coals or a campfire grill for 15 to 20 minutes.
4. Or place foil packet in covered grill on medium-low heat for 7 to 10 minutes.

Nutrition: Calories 668, Sodium 806 mg, Dietary Fiber 23.9 g, Fat 10.9 g, Carbohydrates 111.3 g, Protein 35.6 g

Ranch Chicken Pouches

Ingredients:

- 4 chicken breasts, boneless and skinless
- 2 large potatoes
- 1 onion, chopped
- 1 green pepper, chopped
- 3 carrots, chopped
- 2 celery stalks, chopped
- 4 tablespoons Ranch dressing
- Heavy-duty aluminum foil – 4 pieces of 18" x 24"

Preparation: 10 minutes | Cooking: 50 minutes | Servings: 4

Directions:

1. Boil potatoes for 10 minutes.
2. While potatoes are boiling, chop all ingredients for packets.
3. Cut chicken into bite-size cubes. Drain water from potatoes and cut them into 3/4" cubes.
4. Spray each piece of foil with non-stick cooking spray.
5. Place a chicken breast in the center of each section of foil.
6. Add 1/4 of each of the rest of the ingredients on top of chicken.
7. Pour one tablespoon of Ranch dressing over ingredients on each packet.

8. Fold the foil loosely to form a tent packet, folding and crimping seams tightly.
9. Place foil packet on hot coals or a campfire grill for 30 to 40 minutes. Or place foil packet in covered grill on medium-low heat for 20 to 22 minutes.

Nutrition: Calories 701, Sodium 864 mg, Dietary Fiber 23.2 g, Fat 18.2 g, Carbohydrates 93.5 g, Protein 40.7 g

Retro Baked Mac and Cheese

Ingredients:

- 2 tablespoons butter
- 1 onion, chopped fine
- 4 cups cooked macaroni
- 2 cups whole milk, warmed
- 1 lb. Grated cheese: cheddar, Monterey Jack, or Havarti
- 2 cups broccoli pieces
- 1/4 cup white wine (optional)
- Dash of nutmeg
- Sliced pre-cooked sausage or hotdogs
- 1 cup of potato chips, crumbled
- Salt, to taste
- Pepper, to taste
- Chopped parsley, for garnish
- Ketchup or hot sauce

Preparation: 10 minutes | Cook time: 30 minutes | Servings: 4 to 6

Directions:

1. Heat butter for 30 seconds on medium heat, then add chopped onion and sauté, stirring until beginning to get translucent about 4 minutes.

2. Add milk and stir with a wooden spoon while gently simmering.

3. Add dash of nutmeg and stir.

4. Add grated cheese, putting aside 1 cup for later.

5. When cheese is melted into the milk, add cooked macaroni, broccoli and sausage.

6. Remove from heat and stir well.

7. Sprinkle the rest of the cheese on top, and add crumbled potato chips.

8. Bake at 350°f until the top is brown, about 20 minutes.

9. Serve immediately, sprinkled with parsley.

Nutrition: Calories 499, Sodium 373 mg, Dietary fiber 3.1 g, Fat 22.2 g, Carbohydrates 52.2 g, Protein 20.9 g

Jazzy Spanish Torta

Ingredients:

- 1-tablespoon olive oil
- 1-tablespoon butter
- 2 cloves garlic, minced
- 1 onion, chopped fine
- 2 cups assorted chopped vegetables of your choice
- Red chili flakes
- 1-teaspoon herbs de Provence
- 6 eggs, whisked
- 1/2 cup crumbled goat or feta cheese.
- Salt, to taste
- Pepper, to taste
- Chopped parsley, minced, for garnish

Directions:

1. Heat oil and butter for 30 seconds on medium heat, then add chopped onion and garlic and stir.
2. Cover and continue to cook on medium heat for about 3 - 4 minutes until beginning to get translucent. Stir every minute to prevent burning.
3. Add your chopped vegetables in the following order, browning and stirring between each addition: mushrooms, squash, tomatoes.
4. Whisk eggs with spices and herbs and salt.

95

5. Pour over vegetables.

6. Sprinkle cheese on top.

7. Cover pot and bake in oven for 20 minutes at 350°f. Remove from oven, check that eggs look golden and cooked, and the sides lightly browned.

8. Serve with green salad and bread.

Nutrition: Calories 142, Sodium 243 mg, Dietary Fiber 0.4 g, Fat 11.3 g, Carbohydrates 2.9 g, Protein 7.6 g

Jumble-sale Jambalaya

Ingredients:

- 2 tablespoons olive oil
- 4 cloves garlic, chopped fine
- 1 onion, chopped fine
- 2 cups chopped tomatoes
- 2 cups chopped okra
- 2 cups chopped peppers: red, yellow or green
- 1 cup chopped celery
- 1 jalapeño pepper, seeded and chopped
- 4 chicken thighs or legs; or 2 breasts, cut in halves
- 1/2 lb. Baby shrimp
- 1 smoked ham hock
- 2 spicy (cajun or andouille) sausages
- 1 small can tomato paste
- 4 cups broth of choice
- 4 cups hot water, plus more as needed
- 2 cups white rice, rinsed
- 1/2 teaspoon cayenne pepper,
- 1/2 teaspoon chili powder
- 1/2 teaspoon red pepper flakes
- Salt, to taste
- Pepper, to taste

Preparation: 20 minutes | Cook time: 50 minutes | Servings: 6 to 8

Directions:

1. Heat oil for 30 seconds on medium heat, then add chopped garlic, chopped onion and stir. Cover and continue to cook on medium heat for about 5-6 minutes until beginning to get translucent. Stir every two minutes to prevent burning.

2. Add your vegetables and spices and stir over heat to brown slightly.

3. Add rice, mix and sauté for a minute.

4. Mix broth, hot water and tomato paste. Pour into pot.

5. Making sure the mixture is covered with broth and hot water, throw in your sausages and meats, and stir. Add more hot water if necessary, in beginning.

6. Simmer for 30 minutes.

7. Add peeled shrimp, stir well, and cook for an additional 15 minutes.

8. When rice is soft, turn off heat and let sit for about 10 minutes.

Nutrition: Calories 332, Sodium 686 mg, Dietary Fiber 3.5 g, Fat 7 g, Carbohydrates 3.5 g, Protein 19.8 g

Stuffed Cabbage Osijek Style

Ingredients:

- 2 heads of cabbage
- 1 onion, chopped fine
- 2 cups sauerkraut
- 1 cup rice
- 1/2 lb. ground pork
- 1/2 lb. ground veal or beef
- 2 cups chopped tomatoes
- 1 tablespoon paprika
- 1/2 teaspoon cayenne pepper
- 1/2 cup parsley, minced
- 8 cups or more of hot water
- Salt, to taste
- Pepper, to taste
- Sour cream, for garnish

Preparation: 60 minutes | Cook Time: 90 minutes | Servings: 6 to 8

Directions:

1. Steam heads of cabbage in a large covered pot with about 3 inches of water at bottom, until leaves are soft.
2. Mix the ground meats with the spices, onion, and rice in a bowl. Mix.

3. Taking one cabbage leaf at a time, put 1 tablespoon of meat filling into the soft end, folding the two sides toward the middle like a burrito, and roll towards the root end.

4. Pack tightly at the bottom of pan, folded side down. When one layer is finished, cover with some sauerkraut and add a second layer of stuffed cabbage leaves.

5. Keep placing layers of the stuffed cabbage leaves and sauerkraut packed tightly until you have used up all of the meat and cabbage.

6. Place a ceramic dinner plate over the stuffed cabbages to keep them from floating.

7. Cover completely with hot water.

8. Simmer for one hour or more, until rice is tender and meat filling is fully cooked.

9. To serve, put two or three stuffed leaves in a bowl, place some of the sauerkraut on the side, and add a big dollop of sour cream on top.

Nutrition: Calories 243, Sodium 332 mg, Dietary Fiber 7.1 g, Fat 3.8 g, Carbohydrates 34.2 g, Protein 19.4 g

Papa's Chicken Paprikash

Ingredients:

- 2 tablespoons olive oil
- 2 onions, chopped fine
- 2 cups tomatoes, chopped
- 1 whole chicken, cut into pieces; or 3 chicken legs and 3 thighs
- 1 cup flour, placed in shallow bowl
- 4 potatoes, peeled and quartered
- 4 cups broth, chicken or vegetable
- 2 tablespoons paprika
- 1/4 teaspoon chili
- 1 teaspoon salt or to taste
- Black pepper, to taste
- Sour cream, for garnish

Preparation: 15 minutes | Cook Time: 90 minutes | Servings: 4 to 6

Directions:

1. Heat oil for 30 seconds on medium heat, then add chopped onion and stir. Cover and continue to cook on medium heat for about 5-6 minutes until beginning to get translucent. Stir every two minutes to prevent burning.

2. Dredge chicken pieces in flour. Add to onion and brown, turning once. Remove.

3. Add tomato and simmer to soften.

4. Place chicken parts back into pot.

5. Mix broth with paprika, chili and salt. Pour into pot.

6. Add potatoes and simmer covered until chicken meat is coming off the bone, approximately 1 to 1-1/2 hours.

7. Pepper to taste.

8. Serve with a dollop of sour cream on top.

Nutrition: Calories 411, Sodium 630 mg, Dietary Fiber 6.7 g, Fat 17.5 g, Carbohydrates 46.3 g, Protein 18.5 g

Faint-worthy Stuffed Eggplant

Ingredients:

- 4 tablespoons olive oil, plus
- 4 cloves garlic, chopped fine
- 1 onion, chopped fine
- 6 to 8 small eggplants
- 1 lb. ground lamb
- 1/2 cup pine nuts, toasted in skillet until browned
- 1/2 cup dried currants
- 2 tablespoons chopped mint, fresh or dried
- Dash chili powder
- Dash saffron, soaked in 1/4 cup warm water
- Salt, to taste
- Pepper, to taste

Preparation: 30 minutes | Cook Time: 60 minutes | Servings: 4 to 6

Directions:

1. Put eggplants on a baking sheet or in a cast iron skillet and broil until they are slightly browned.
2. Prepare the filling – mix the meat with garlic, onion, pine nuts, currants, and spices.
3. Split the eggplants in half lengthwise, and remove the inner part of the flesh leaving a trough for the filling.

Leave at least 1/4-inch of flesh on the inside of the skin.

4. Put spoonful of the filling into the troughs, so that the eggplant is nicely filled.
5. Put olive oil into base of cast iron cooker.
6. Pack the stuffed eggplant halves into the bottom of the pan. You can add layers of the eggplant if necessary, but do it carefully so as not to spill the filling.
7. Cover with chopped tomatoes, add 1 cup of broth to the pot from the side, cover with the lid and bake at 350°F for one hour.
8. Serve with yogurt on the side.

Nutrition: Calories 333, Sodium 88 mg, Dietary Fiber 4.2 g, Fat 22.8 g, Carbohydrates 10 g, Protein 24.1 g

Messy Moussaka

Ingredients:

- 1/4 cup olive oil
- 4 cloves garlic, chopped fine
- 1 onion, chopped fine
- 2 large eggplants, sliced into half inch slices, lengthwise.
- 1 lb. ground lamb or beef
- 1/2 cup pine nuts
- 1/2 cup currants
- 2 cups chopped tomatoes
- 1 cup tomato sauce
- 1/2 teaspoon dried or fresh mint, minced
- 1/4 teaspoon cayenne pepper
- 1/2 teaspoon nutmeg
- Salt, to taste
- Pepper, to taste

Béchamel sauce:

- 4 tablespoons salted butter
- 4 tablespoons flour
- 2 cups whole milk
- Dash of nutmeg
- Dash of pepper
- 1/2 cup grated white cheese, such as cheddar

Preparation: 30 minutes | Cook Time: 40 minutes | Servings: 4 to 6

Directions:

Make béchamel sauce:

1. Scald milk and put aside.
2. Melt butter in casserole, add flour, and mix constantly for two minutes to thicken. Add scalded milk, nutmeg, salt, pepper, and cook, but do not boil. Stir while simmering, about 5 minutes.
3. Add grated cheese, mix thoroughly over heat until well blended, and put aside.

Meat and Eggplant Layers:

1. Mix meat with garlic, onion, currants, pine nuts, herbs, and spices.
2. Brush cooking pot with light film of olive oil.
3. Put a layer of the eggplant slices, tightly packed and brushed with olive oil, on the bottom.
4. Cover eggplant with meat mixture.
5. Add a thin layer of the béchamel sauce.
6. Repeat layering of eggplant, olive oil, filling and béchamel sauce.
7. Make sure the final layer on top is just eggplant slices.
8. Cover with the rest of your béchamel sauce.

9. Place in oven and bake uncovered for 40 minutes at 350°F; or until top is nicely browned and interior filling is bubbling.

Nutrition: Calories 509, Sodium 408 mg, Dietary Fiber 8.2 g, Fat 33.4 g, Carbohydrates 26.5 g, Protein 29.6 g

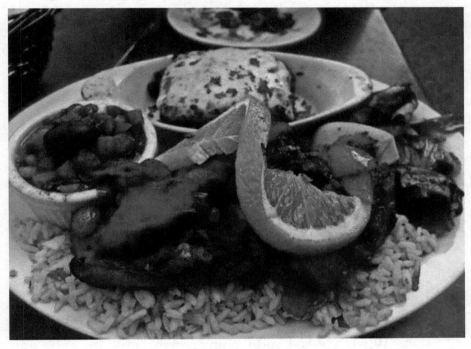

Polenta Derventa

Ingredients:

- 2 cups cornmeal
- 8 cups broth, either vegetable or chicken
- 4 strips bacon
- 1 cup sour cream
- 1/2 cup minced parsley

Preparation: 10 minutes | Cook Time: 40 minutes | Servings: 4 to 6

Directions:

1. Cook bacon in pot, removing when becoming crisp. Put aside.
2. Add cornmeal to bacon fat, stir well over heat for a minute.
3. Add broth, stir, and cook over medium heat.
4. Simmer and stir often until thick, about 30 minutes.
5. When cooked, add sour cream, mix in well, and sprinkle with parsley.
6. Serve.

Nutrition: Calories 351, Sodium 348 mg, Dietary Fiber 3.1 g, Fat 16.6 g, Carbohydrates 34.6 g, Protein: 15.8 g

Lazy Lasagna with Ground Beef or Vegetables

Ingredients:

- 8 - 10 tablespoons olive oil or as needed
- 1 box lasagna strips, uncooked
- 4 cups tomato Sauce
- 2 cups tomatoes, chopped
- 6 cloves garlic, minced
- 1/2 cup parsley, minced
- 2 cups mushrooms, sliced and sautéed
- 2 cups ground beef, sautéed
- 2 tablespoons rosemary, dried; or fresh minced
- 1 lb. mozzarella, grated or sliced

Preparation: 20 minutes | Cook Time: 45 minutes| Servings: 4 to 6

Directions:

1. Mix meat with herbs, mushrooms, tomato and garlic
2. Place 2 tablespoons of olive oil at base of pot and spread evenly.
3. Place strips of uncooked pasta; cover with more oil, then the meat (or veg) mixture.
4. Cover this with some cheese.
5. Pour some tomato sauce on top.

6. Repeat this process until you have layered all the pasta and filling and most of the cheese.

7. Pour remaining tomato sauce over the top.

8. Cover with remaining cheese.

9. Bake uncovered at 350°F for 45 minutes, or until pasta is tender.

Nutrition: Calories 681, Sodium 150 mg, Dietary Fiber 5.7 g, Fat 48.2 g, Carbohydrates 22.6 g, Protein 42.2 g

Lightning Source UK Ltd.
Milton Keynes UK
UKHW021400070521
383304UK00001B/42